# A LITTLE BOOK OF DOCTORS' RULES

# A LITTLE BOOK OF DOCTORS' RULES

*edited by*

## CLIFTON K. MEADOR, M.D.

*Philadelphia*
HANLEY & BELFUS, INC.

*St. Louis • Baltimore • Boston • Chicago • London • Philadelphia • Sydney • Toronto*
MOSBY–YEAR BOOK, INC.

Published by HANLEY & BELFUS, INC., 210 S. 13th Street,
Philadelphia, PA 19107. (215) 546-7293; 800-962-1892.

North American and worldwide sales and distribution:
Mosby–Year Book, Inc., 11830 Westline Industrial Drive, St. Louis, MO 63146.
In Canada: The C. V. Mosby Company, Ltd., 5240 Finch Avenue East, Unit 1,
Scarborough, Ontario M1S 5A2, Canada.

*Designed by Adrianne Onderdonk Dudden*

A LITTLE BOOK OF DOCTORS' RULES          ISBN 1-56053-061-8
© 1992 by Clifton K. Meador, M.D.

Last digit is the print number: 9 8 7 6 5 4 3 2 1

## PREFACE

I have often thought there should be a set of rules for the practice of medicine. In medical school, residency, and later, I hoped to find such a collection. I believed it would assist me in developing my skills as a physician. I never found one one that met my needs. Of course I read the aphorisms of Hippocrates, Osler, and others. All were dated and, from a practical sense, outdated.

Through the years I heard or read concise and useful ideas about the practice of medicine. I made mental notes, testing these clinical notions in my teaching and practice.

This book is my effort to compile, in no order other than the sequence in which I recalled and recorded them, these rules, observations, and helpful tips. I hope they will be useful, especially to those just entering the study of medicine.

There are three tests that I have attempted to apply to each of the rules:

*First,* a good rule makes intuitive sense. It has a ring of truth.

*Second,* a valid rule has been observed to be helpful in its application or harmful in its violation.

*Third,* a sound rule is stated in a manner that allows affirmation or refutation by direct, systematic observations of others. This last consideration fulfills the important and essential potential for being scientific.

Although I did not make it a requirement, I have also selected rules that expose the humorous side of the practice of medicine. I trust I have not offended too many with this effort. It is almost (but not quite) a rule that we physicians take ourselves far too seriously, sometimes forgetting we are human. I have found the practice of medicine to be a highly entertaining activity, and I wish to convey some sense of that in these rules.

My fascination has always been more with the nature of the practice of medicine than with its actual practice. I have often wondered what it is that constitutes the real stuff of the practice of medicine. What are its essential elements? What is it we do that is helpful? What do we do that is harmful? Is there a way to codify and describe these necessary elements? Can we tease out the unspoken and unwritten rules by which we operate and which determine our behavior and make us physicians? Can we begin to explore the hazy art of the practice of medicine in some systematic way? Can we create a science of the art of the practice of medicine?

I have two final comments. First, the nearly random presentation of the rules has troubled some of my colleagues. However, I find it pleasing because it conveys the unpredictable and at times chaotic nature of the interaction between a given physician and a given patient, especially the first encounter at the level of primary care. Besides, I thought an unsystematic arrangement would pique your interest as a reader in a way that a highly structured order would not.

Finally, because this is an initial effort, I hope readers will join me in making explicit their own implicit little rules by which they enjoy the practice of medicine. Feel free to send in your own rule or a modification or comment about any in this book for inclusion in the next edition. A suggestion form is provided at the end of the book.

Clifton K. Meador, M.D.

# ACKNOWLEDGMENTS

In early drafts of the rules, I considered giving separate credit for each of the rules. I have rejected this notion for several reasons. First, a good rule should stand on its own and not rely on any authority. If it is a valid rule, it does not matter who introduced it. Second, although I thought I created some of the rules, I could not be sure. After a while it is difficult to separate one's own thoughts from the accumulation of the thoughts of others. Over the years I have read extensively and therefore would have to list far too many sources if I were to attempt to give credit for all the rules I have drawn from the literature.

The final reason I am not giving separate credit for each rule is that I do not recall the source of all the rules. I will, however, try to give credit where I do recall special input that was formative.

From my readings, I will begin with Hippocrates then mention Galen and continue with Descartes, Bacon, Sydenham, Laennec, the Hunters, Bernard, Cushing and on to Sir William Osler, whose writings and aphorisms no doubt stimulated me to update many of his ideas and guiding principles. Lewis Thomas and John Stone cover many of the rules in their prose. Garrison's *History of Medicine* was a rich source for many of the rules. And then there is the continuing rich medical literature.

My teachers and mentors directly influenced the creation of the rules in many ways. All were superior physicians. Tinsley Harrison taught the value of listening, dissecting out the details of symptoms, and, specifically, the value of having the patient keep a diary. Rudolph Kampmeier taught the systematic gathering of clinical information and the primacy of the history over all other sources of clinical data. John Shapiro showed me the way to correlate symptoms with pathological findings. Elliot Newman pushed me to doubt and question. Robert F. Loeb, my chief during house officer training, generated most of the rules of therapy and those related to the prudent and careful use of drugs. Grant Liddle, my mentor in endocrinology, instilled the importance of measurable data and the essential need for direct observation. David Rogers, my chief in later residency, taught me how to make careful examinations and observations of patients. Much later, Joseph Sapira taught me how to listen and to facilitate the patient's telling of his story. Bertram Sprofkin taught me accurate neurological observations and the problems from our deteriorating use of the English language.

James Pittman taught me high regard for the literature, medical and other. John Freymann taught me the value of historical perspective. Much, much later, there was Stonewall Stickney, who taught me respect for the efforts of modern psychiatry.

Many friends and colleagues read the early versions of the rules and gave helpful suggestions. Most shared some of their own rules with me, which I now pass on to you. These include Paul Michael MD, Mark Averbuch MD, Philip Felts MD, John Newman MD, Mary Schaffner JD, Kelley Avery MD, William Stoney MD, Barton Campbell MD, Harry Page MD, Al Roach D Pharm, John Dixon MD, Mary Ann Clark, Allen Kaiser MD, John Sergent MD, Clarence Thomas MD, Mitzi Sprouse RN, Curtis G. Tribble MD, Seth Cooper MD, E.E. Anderson MD, Richard M. Zaner PhD, Sister Almeda Golson DC, Sister Elise Beaudreaux DC, and Sister Colette Hanlon SC. I owe special thanks to Rosalie Hammerschmidt Lanius RN, who, while in practice with me, participated in the formation of many of the rules.

Another group of people to whom I owe special thanks are the numerous students, residents, and fellows I have had the privilege of teaching and learning from through the years. Many have unwittingly added rules of their own through their thoughts and actions. Over the course of 30 years I have had the opportunity to observe just about every imaginable helpful and nonhelpful interaction between physician and patient. Many of the rules derive from these observations.

I have also had the good fortune to spend time with many practicing physicians across a wide geographic area over many years. My first opportunity came as Dean of the Medical School of the University of Alabama in Birmingham when I traveled up and down the state for a five-year period. My second was while on sabbatical leave at the University of South Alabama

School of Medicine when I visited over 20 communities on a weekly basis, meeting with physicians and conducting medical educational programs across most of the state of Alabama. In these meetings I met and examined a large number of patients and observed in close detail the practices of many physicians. Many of the pearls of practice I have recorded come from the experiences and wisdom of these physicians. There are too many of them to list, and I have long forgotten which one contributed which thought. I deeply appreciate the chance I had to meet and work with all of these men and women who taught me so much.

And then there are the patients, the center and purpose of all of our learning. There are far too many of them to name, even if I were allowed to do so. I owe special thanks to all the patients who have allowed me to participate in their care.

CKM

**THERE IS NO RULE WITHOUT AN EXCEPTION.**
**MOST RULES CAN BE BROKEN.**

| 1 | Sit down when you talk with patients. |

| 2 | Always examine the part that hurts. Put your hand on the area. |

| 3 | Touch the patient, even if you only shake hands or feel the pulse, especially with old people. |

But not with paranoids.

| 4 | You often have to throw out some result or finding. Choose wisely what you discard. |

5 | There is no blood or urine test to differentiate a well person from a sick one.

6 | The only way to determine if a person is well or sick is to
listen,
look carefully,
ask good questions,
and make a sound clinical decision.

7 | There is no blood or urine test to measure mental function.
There probably never will be.

8 | The good clinician knows what he or she does not know.

9 | If in doubt about dementia, do a mental status evaluation.

| 10 | Learn to do a thorough mental status evaluation.

Do it as you go along.

Fill it in later:

    mood,
    affect,
    attitude,
    appearance,
    disorganized vs. organized,
    rapport,
    speech content,
    delusions, hallucinations,
    judgment,
    memory, recent and remote

| 11 | Know which abnormality you are going to follow during treatment.

Pick something you can measure.

**12** If there is no abnormality to follow,
do not treat with drugs or surgery.

**13** If a drug is not working, stop it.

**14** If a drug is working, keep it up.
This applies to patients with chronic conditions.

**15** In acutely ill patients who are being treated, do not change
anything if the patient is getting better.

**16** Change only one drug at a time.

**17** Use the smallest number of drugs possible.

**18** Stop all drugs if possible.
If impossible, stop as many as possible.

**19** Be very careful if you decide to treat a drug reaction with another drug.

A better rule:
   Never treat a drug reaction with another drug unless the second drug is a proven antidote for the first.

**20** There is no such thing as an organ-specific drug.

All drugs work throughout the body.

**21** Do not get your drug information exclusively from drug salesmen.

**22** Use as few drugs as possible in your practice.
Know these in detail.

23   When a patient comes to you taking drugs you do not know, read about them—
and then stop as many as possible.

24   It is usually not worth the time and emotional drain to try to stop fat women from taking thyroid replacement agents or thin women from taking vitamin B12 injections.

25   It is usually not worth the time and effort to try to stop older patients from taking laxatives.

26   Be wary of patients who are too complimentary of you as a physician, especially on the first visit.

27   You cannot be everybody's physician.

28 Learn to distinguish those patients for whom you can be their physician from those for whom you cannot.

Refer the latter to another physician.
Do it sooner than later.

29 Patients with factitious disease (secretly self-inflicted disease) do not remain with the physician who makes the diagnosis.

30 When you are listening to a patient, do not do anything else. Just listen.

31 The interview is the beginning of treatment.

32 Read Ian Stevenson's *The Diagnostic Interview.**

* Stevenson I: The Diagnostic Interview. New York, Harper and Row, 1971.

**33** Tell patients to remove the foil from a suppository before insertion.

**34** Read Charles E. Odegaard's *Dear Doctor: A Personal Letter to a Physician,** especially the appendices.

**35** The absence of a demonstrable medical disease in a symptomatic patient does not automatically establish a diagnosis of mental illness.

Contrariwise, the presence of a demonstrable medical disease in a symptomatic patient does not automatically rule out mental illness.

Violation of both rules is common and a source of great error.

* Odegaard CE: Dear Doctor: A Personal Letter to a Physician. Menlo Park, CA, Henry J. Kaiser Family Foundation, 1986.

**36** If you do not know what is wrong with a patient after you have taken a history, then take another history.

If you still do not know, take a third history.

If you do not know then, you probably never will.

**37** Never tell a symptomatic patient, "Don't worry. It's all in your head."*

**38** Never tell a symptomatic patient, "There is nothing wrong with you."

It is demeaning and insulting.

**39** A patient under the age of 50 with several symptoms probably has only one disease.

* Joseph Sapira tells the story of a chairman of psychiatry who broke his leg in a skiing accident. After the x-rays were developed, the orthopedic surgeon said, "Don't worry, it's all in your body."

40    A patient over the age of 50 with several symptoms probably has more than one disease.

41    When you do not know what a patient has, do not say, "I don't know what you have."

Say, "I don't know what you have . . . YET."

42    When:

     the patient has multiple complaints,

     you do not know what the patient has,

     the workup has been thorough but negative, and

     you suspect there is no demonstrable medical illness to
        explain the symptoms;

Say, "I KNOW what you DO NOT HAVE."

Then slowly list every disease that you know the patient does NOT have. Be sure to include a long and tedious list of every known disease you can think of.

Do this until you are sure the patient is bored.

43 When you are telling patients what they DO NOT HAVE, be sure to include those diseases most feared and especially those that killed close members of the family. Do this only if you are sure you have excluded those diseases.

44 Never reassure a new patient with multiple chronic complaints too early about the absence of a specific disease.
Wait a few days. He or she will believe you then.

45 When taking a detailed drug history, start with the drugs taken today,
then the day before,
then the day before that.

46 Most office patients get well with or without you.

47 Most people are healthy and will live long lives.

THE LAW OF PREVALENCE.*

Under the LAW OF PREVALENCE, false-positive values are the diagnostic pitfall with outpatients in primary care practice.

When a patient is not sick or has come only for a checkup, discard and repeat positive test results.

Under the LAW OF PREVALENCE, false-negative values are the diagnostic pitfall with the critically ill.

When a patient is very ill, discard and repeat important negative test results.

---

* The equation that states the LAW OF PREVALENCE is:

$$\text{Predictive Value (Positive Test)} = \frac{\text{prevalence} \times \text{Se}}{(\text{prevalence} \times \text{Se}) + (1-\text{prevalence})(1-\text{Sp})}$$

Where Se = sensitivity
Sp = specificity

From its position in the equation, one can readily see the power of prevalence.

| 49 | Drugs should make patients feel better, not worse.

| 50 | If a drug makes a patient feel worse, stop it and find a suitable alternative.

| 51 | Be wary of patients who smile:
when they describe pain,
or severe symptoms,
or misfortunes in life,
or the failures of doctors to help, so far.

| 52 | Learn to watch people's faces.

| 53 | Learn to watch people's nostril size.

| 54 | Learn to watch the lower lip and then the upper lip.

| 55 | Learn to watch the skin color of the face. |

| 56 | Notice the change in respiratory rate as you discuss different subjects with your patients. |

The top edge of the shoulders moves with each inhalation.

| 57 | A very fat person who is losing weight probably has a disease, even if he says he is on a diet. |

| 58 | Give the patient permission to discuss unusual or deviant behavior. Do this in a specific manner: |

If you think a patient may be abusing laxatives, say, "Some people take only a tablespoon of milk of magnesia a day, some take 2 or 3 bottles a day. How much do you take?"

If you think a patient is abusing enemas, say, "Some patients I know take an enema once a month, others several times a day. How often do you?"

**59** You do not have to like a patient,
but it sure helps.

If the dislike is severe,
the patient may have a serious personality disorder or may be
acting out an aspect of yourself that you despise or disown.

If you still do not like a patient after three visits, refer him or
her to someone else.

**60** All patients will lie about something.
Some will lie about everything.

**61** Being a physician is a high privilege.
Do not abuse it.

**62** The medical school curriculum is a poor format for learning
anything about life.

63  Respect everyone you meet, especially those who work at
menial jobs in the hospital.

They make it possible for you to be a physician.

64  The odds of you as a physician
committing suicide,
getting addicted,
getting divorced,
becoming an alcoholic, or
going off the deep end are very high.
Find out why.

65  Know those things you can change.

Know those things you cannot change.

Develop the wisdom to tell the difference.

| 66 | Do not refer to patients as diseases.
Do not say, "the gallbladder in room _____ ."
   or the "cardiac"
   or the "kidney failure"
   or the "chronic lunger."

| 67 | Always be careful of hysterical patients.

They can have several diseases.

| 68 | Just because you know a lot of physiology, biochemistry, and anatomy does not mean you know anything about life or people.

Let your patients and other people teach you.

| 69 | Learn something from every patient you meet.

**70** There is no such thing as an uninteresting patient.
They are all fascinating in some way.
Discover what that is.

**71** If you do not like clinical medicine, get out of it today.

**72** Learn to say "No" tactfully.
Just say "No."

**73** Say "No" at least once every day.

**74** Never explain why you are saying "No."

**75** Do not discuss your personal life with patients.
If you feel an urge to do that, make some new friends or
reconnect with your family.

| 76 | Be wary of seductive patients.
Learn how to deal with them in a straightforward manner.
If the behavior continues, refer the patient to another physician.

| 77 | Never, ever, have a sexual relationship with a patient or with an office employee.

| 78 | Do not treat *acute* anxiety with drugs, except in real emergencies.

| 79 | Depression comes in two forms:

There is little "d" depression. We all get that. It is a part of grief or worry. It passes. Do not treat little "d" depression with drugs.

There is big "D" DEPRESSION. It is a disease that requires antidepressant drugs, with the dosage adjusted carefully to the level needed.

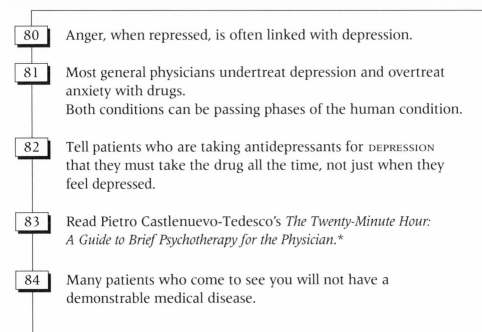

80   Anger, when repressed, is often linked with depression.

81   Most general physicians undertreat depression and overtreat anxiety with drugs.
     Both conditions can be passing phases of the human condition.

82   Tell patients who are taking antidepressants for DEPRESSION that they must take the drug all the time, not just when they feel depressed.

83   Read Pietro Castlenuevo-Tedesco's *The Twenty-Minute Hour: A Guide to Brief Psychotherapy for the Physician.*\*

84   Many patients who come to see you will not have a demonstrable medical disease.

\* Castlenuevo-Tedesco P: The Twenty-Minute Hour. Boston, Little, Brown and Company, 1965.

**85** The progress of many symptoms (for example, pain) can be followed by use of a self-rating scale from 0 to 10.

**86** Prevalence is to the diagnostic process what gravity is to the planetary system.

It has the power of a physical law.

Above all other factors, it controls the accuracy of the diagnostic process.

**87** Prevalence of serious disease varies widely according to the site of practice.

It is low in community or family practice,
high in a referral diagnostic center,
extremely high in a referral critical care unit.

**88** Read *Beyond Normality* by Galen and Gambino.*

**89** If you are going into a career in academic medicine, spend at least one year away from an academic center in the private practice of medicine.

**90** If you are going into private practice, spend at least one year in an academic medical center doing research.

Learn one small area in great depth.
It will give you respect for scientific knowledge.

**91** Choose and buy one of the standard textbooks of medicine.
Buy the latest edition whenever it is published.
Do this for the rest of your career.

* Galen RS, Gambino SR: Beyond Normality: The Predictive Value and Efficiency of Medical Diagnoses. New York, John Wiley and Sons, 1975.

| 92 | Subscribe to *JAMA* or *The New England Journal of Medicine*. Read it every week. If you do not read it, at least scan it. |

| 93 | Read the chapter in a standard textbook of medicine about each new disease or symptom you encounter. Do this the rest of your career. |

| 94 | If you do not know what a sick patient has after a thorough workup, get a consultation.

If you do not know after the first consultation, get another one.

Then, if you do not know, refer the patient to a well-known medical center.

If you practice in a medical center and still do not know, refer the patient to another medical center. |

| 95 | Consultants should discuss recommendations only with the referring physician and not with the patient.

This rule is no longer followed.
It should be.

| 96 | Some patients are beyond existing medical knowledge.

| 97 | Some patients are beyond all knowledge.

| 98 | Some diseases are not treatable,
but all patients can be given care.

| 99 | Untreatable diseases should not be treated unless the patient agrees to be included in an experimental protocol.

| 100 | Learn when and when not to call a surgeon.

| 101 | Severe, acute abdominal pain always requires a surgical consultation. |
| --- | --- |
| 102 | A good surgeon evaluating acute abdominal pain is equivalent to a highly sensitive and specific laboratory test. |
| 103 | An acute surgical abdomen is when a good surgeon says it is an acute surgical abdomen.<br><br>There is no other test for it. |
| 104 | Develop a list of physicians you trust and respect, nurture your relationship with them, and contact them about difficult cases.<br><br>Select one in each of the specialties and call them as often as you need. |

105 There are only three ways to answer a question:
I don't know.
I don't know, but I'll guess.
I know.

106 If you need time to think, ask older patients to describe their bowel habits.

107 Almost all diseased patients look sick, talk sick, and act sick.

A few diseased patients look well, talk well, and act well.

A few people without disease can look sick, talk sick, and act sick.

Be careful.

108 Whatever subject the patient is most comfortable discussing is probably not the real trouble.

| 109 | Symptoms attributable to medical diseases tend to get better or worse.

Physical symptoms attributable to psychological disorders tend to stay about the same over time.

| 110 | Time is the greatest diagnostician.

Use it wisely.

| 111 | Most patients can tell you why they got sick.

| 112 | Most patients can tell you what their sickness is.

| 113 | If a patient gets sick taking multiple drugs, one or more of the drugs is causing the symptoms.

Stop the drugs and observe.

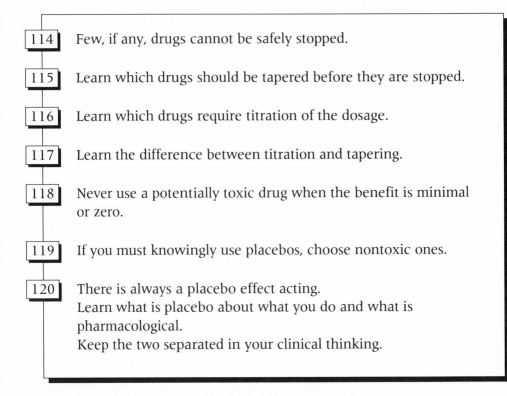

114     Few, if any, drugs cannot be safely stopped.

115     Learn which drugs should be tapered before they are stopped.

116     Learn which drugs require titration of the dosage.

117     Learn the difference between titration and tapering.

118     Never use a potentially toxic drug when the benefit is minimal or zero.

119     If you must knowingly use placebos, choose nontoxic ones.

120     There is always a placebo effect acting.
Learn what is placebo about what you do and what is pharmacological.
Keep the two separated in your clinical thinking.

121 | All patients—those with PhDs in psychology, those who hold high public offices, the illiterate, and the ignorant—want magic from you.

Magic does not require pills or surgery.

122 | Read Jerome Frank's *Persuasion and Healing*.\*

123 | If all you listen to are symptoms, then all you will hear from your patients are symptoms.
All of your patients will have symptoms.

If you can listen to a variety of subjects, then fewer and fewer of your patients will have symptoms.
Some of your patients will stop having symptoms.

---

\* Frank J: Persuasion and Healing: A Comparative Study of Psychotherapy. New York, Schocken Books, 1974.

124   Like it or not, there is a little "witch doctor" operating in all physicians.

Use that skill wisely and only for the benefit of your patients.

125   There are three kinds of patients.
1. Those who believe every word you say and do everything you suggest.

    Be careful what you say and suggest.
2. Those who reflect on what you say, wonder why you said it, ask you questions, and then make up their own minds about what they do.

    Answer all their questions.
3. Those who disagree with everything you say, oppose every suggestion you make, and state that nothing will help them.

    Preface every suggestion you make by saying you do not think the treatment will work. Lead them to argue that the treatment will work and it will.

Learn to deal with all three kinds of patients.

**126** For patients with acute, severe, incapacitating pain, use enough narcotics to relieve pain. Do this intravenously until the patient is comfortable.

**127** For patients with chronic pain, no matter how severe, do not use narcotics unless the patient has a terminal disease. Then use all that is needed to relieve pain.

**128** Most patients with chronic headaches do not know how to use aspirin correctly. Here is one method:

With the first inkling of a headache, take three aspirin.

Half an hour later, unless the pain is abating, take two more.

One hour later, unless the pain is much better, take one more.

It is a rare headache that fails to respond to this schedule.

**129** Teach patients to be well, not sick.

**130** If you catch yourself thinking a patient might have either hyperthyroidism or hypothyroidism, then the patient does not have either.

**131** There are two types of fat people:

Those who are fat from childhood.
Those who gain weight later in life.

There is a very different prognosis for sustained weight loss for the two types.

**132** The weight and height tables are not verities.

There are tall people and there are short people.
There are heavy people and there are thin people.
There are endomorphs, ectomorphs, and mesomorphs.

Everybody has to be one thing or another.

**133** Let patients ramble for at least 5 minutes when you first see them.
You will learn a lot.

**134** Some people have fast brains, others have slow brains.
Adjust your thinking to the pace of the patient.

**135** Listen for what the patient is NOT telling you.

**136** Never appear shocked by anything a patient tells you.

**137** Read Jay Haley's *Uncommon Therapy: The Psychiatric Techniques of Milton H. Erickson, M.D.*\*
This is an account of Milton Erickson's therapeutic genius.

\* Haley J: Uncommon Therapy: The Psychiatric Techniques of Milton H. Erickson, M.D. New York, W.W. Norton and Company, 1973.

THE SHOCKING WILD GUESS METHOD

For the patient who repeatedly says, "I can't talk about . . . *that*":

If the question was about the husband, you make a wild guess that he is a felon or some equally startling notion.

If the question was about a child, you make a wild guess that he tortures pets with fire or something equally abhorrent to a parent.

There are two possible results with this method.

Your guess will be correct and you will appear clairvoyant, permitting the patient to talk more freely about the taboo.

or

Your guessed answer will be so much worse than reality, the patient will feel relieved and more comfortable about telling the truth to prove you incorrect.

The taboo is defused either way.

FOR ADVANCED STUDENTS ONLY

For those rare patients who have multiple chronic symptoms and who jump from one symptom to another, here is one way to contain them:

> Put labels on several chairs in the exam room.
> Label one "head," another "legs," still another "chest," and yet another "stomach."
>
> Then say, "I am confused with all your symptoms. It will help me to keep your symptoms straight if you will sit in the appropriate chair when you talk about each one."

After a few chair changes, patients often begin to talk about what is really bothering them. They may drop all mention of symptoms.

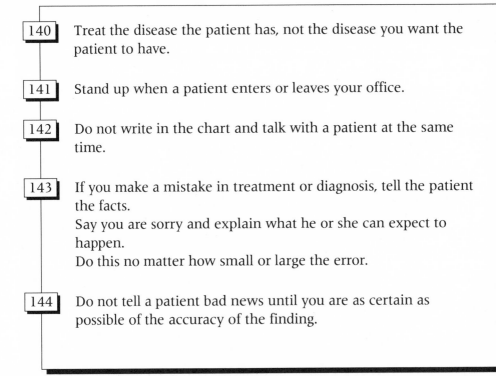

140    Treat the disease the patient has, not the disease you want the patient to have.

141    Stand up when a patient enters or leaves your office.

142    Do not write in the chart and talk with a patient at the same time.

143    If you make a mistake in treatment or diagnosis, tell the patient the facts.
Say you are sorry and explain what he or she can expect to happen.
Do this no matter how small or large the error.

144    Do not tell a patient bad news until you are as certain as possible of the accuracy of the finding.

145 If you are doing a screening test that has a high probability of being falsely positive, tell the patient ahead of time that you may need to get a second specimen and sometimes a third one before you can be sure of the results.

If the first test is positive, do the appropriate second test but do not discuss the results of the first test with the patient.

Let the patient know the test is complicated and subject to variation *before* you order it.

146 Never order a test unless the result will help you direct the treatment or make a difference in what you tell a patient.

147 Do not go on "fishing expeditions" for diseases that are not dictated by the history, the physical examination, or the circumstances of the case.

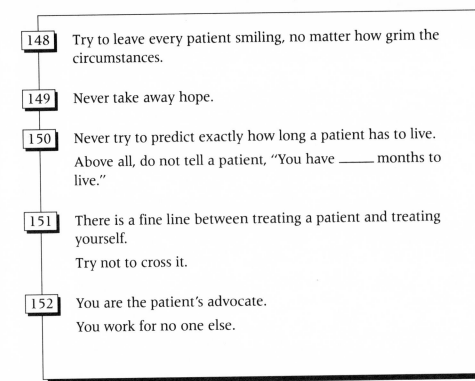

**148** Try to leave every patient smiling, no matter how grim the circumstances.

**149** Never take away hope.

**150** Never try to predict exactly how long a patient has to live.

Above all, do not tell a patient, "You have _____ months to live."

**151** There is a fine line between treating a patient and treating yourself.

Try not to cross it.

**152** You are the patient's advocate.

You work for no one else.

153 After you make a diagnosis and begin treatment, if the patient does not get better, be willing to throw out your first diagnosis and start over.

Do this in your thinking before you tell your patient.

154 With an undiagnosed seriously ill patient, there is probably a physician somewhere who will know what the patient has.

Find that physician.

155 If you enter the hospital room of a married man and notice a woman quietly pass you, avoiding all eye contact, it is probably the man's mistress.

156 With seriously or terminally ill patients, be wary of kin from afar.

They are often trouble.

**157** Avoid all meetings where ex-wives, present wives, and lovers are present.

Likewise for meetings with husbands, ex-husbands, and lovers.

**158** If a wife refuses to leave the room of her husband and makes every effort to prevent you from talking to him alone, then make sure you do talk to the man alone even if you have to arrange it in the radiology department.

**159** A husband rarely refuses to leave his wife alone with a physician.

Many never even come to the hospital.

**160** Most patients are women.

(Do men worry them sick?)

**161** When a man seeks medical care, there usually is a woman urging him to do it.

Talk with her.

**162** Do not talk to an angry patient about any other subject until you understand the source of his or her anger.

Take as long as necessary to diffuse the anger.

**163** It is all right for a patient to get angry.

**164** It is all right for a patient to cry,
   get depressed,
   laugh,
   hurt,
   or have any other feeling.

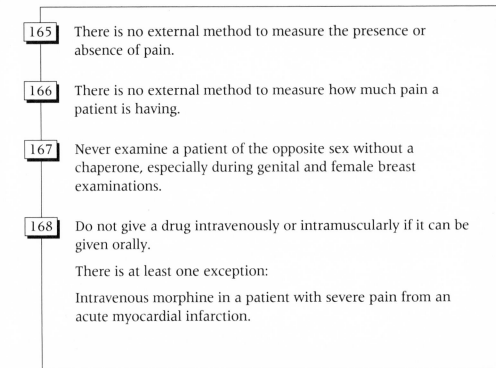

**165** There is no external method to measure the presence or absence of pain.

**166** There is no external method to measure how much pain a patient is having.

**167** Never examine a patient of the opposite sex without a chaperone, especially during genital and female breast examinations.

**168** Do not give a drug intravenously or intramuscularly if it can be given orally.

There is at least one exception:

Intravenous morphine in a patient with severe pain from an acute myocardial infarction.

**169** Rare manifestations of common diseases are more common than common manifestations of rare diseases.

**170** Any juvenile diabetic patient with recurrent admissions for ketoacidosis is omitting insulin until proven otherwise.

Confrontation of this is rarely if ever helpful.
Knowing this, however, can be very helpful.

**171** Any new abnormality that occurs with the administration of a new drug is due to the drug until proved otherwise.

**172** There is no manifestation that cannot be caused by any given drug.

   or

Any drug can do anything.

**173** There are no controlled studies of patients taking more than four drugs and very few of patients taking three.

Any patient on more than four drugs is beyond medical science.

**174** The likelihood of an adverse drug reaction rises exponentially with any increase in the number of drugs administered.

**175** If the patient is a man and there are several women present in the room when you enter, never guess which one is the wife.

And never ever guess if one of them is the mother.
She may be the man's wife.

**176** Some patients have a need to be sick.
Do not deny them that need.

**177** Illness behavior attracts attention.
All illness has some secondary gain.

**178** Tincture of time is frequently the best medicine.

**179** Physical symptoms due to medical diseases either get worse or get better.

Physical symptoms attributable to a psychological origin do not change very much over time.

**180** The absence of a reported specific toxicity of a drug does not mean it cannot or does not occur.

**181** Drug reactions can be unique to a single patient.

**182** Some diseases are idiosyncratic and peculiar to one patient.

**183** Screening for the presence of a disease in a well person is a very different process from documenting the presence of the same disease in a sick one.

**184** When you evaluate seriously ill patients, shape your list of possibilities to those diseases that are treatable, even if they are rare.

**185** Never let a patient die with a rare but treatable disease.

**186** Do not worry about missing diagnoses of untreatable diseases.

**187** A middle-aged man who suddenly develops what appears to be a character disorder, or a dysphasia, or some new behavior has a brain tumor until proven otherwise.

**188** Absence of clinical evidence is not evidence for its absence.

189 | Learn to perform a detailed and thorough neurological examination.

190 | Become an expert on what is and what is not a Babinski response.

It will serve you well.

191 | A sign is either "present" or "absent."
Signs are never "positive" or "negative."

192 | Avoid use of the terms "negative" or "normal" in describing a physical examination.
Never use "essentially" or "basically" normal.

Describe what you see, hear, or feel and what you do not.

193 | Use the English language correctly and concisely.

| 194 | No verbal presentation of a case should ever take more than five minutes.

Longer presentations mean you do not know what you are talking about.

| 195 | Do not say "In my experience" until you have been in practice at least ten years. Even then, use the term sparingly or not at all.

| 196 | When caring for a very sick patient, doubt all results of all tests.

| 197 | Learn to check for the name of your patient on all laboratory and other test results.

Reports and results get switched.

| 198 | Learn to look at all x-ray/imaging studies personally. Make a habit of reviewing all abnormal or questionable findings with a radiologist.

199 Human biology and clinical medicine are not the same discipline.

Human biologists and clinicians use very different thought processes.

200 The pathophysiology of the diagnosed disease should explain the patient's symptoms.

If it does not, you either have the wrong diagnosis or you are missing a second disease that could explain the symptoms.

201 Learn what treatments are futile.

202 If a treatment is futile, do not use it.

203 Old people are fragile and decompensate easily.
Work them up gently.
Treat them carefully with drugs, if drugs are necessary.

204 | Most old people do better and feel better when they stop taking all drugs.

205 | A lot of what is called aging is simply disuse and inactivity.

Gently push old patients to stretch all their muscles daily and go for daily walks.

206 | Make a list of lethal but treatable diseases.
Make a vow that you will never miss a diagnosis of any of them.
Be sure to include the following:

Diabetic ketoacidosis or any acidosis
Hyperosmolar states
Meningitis (bacterial, fungal, or tuberculous)
Cryptic blood loss
Thyrotoxicosis
Addison's disease
Toxic shock

Rocky Mountain spotted fever
Dehydration
Hypoxemia
Obstructive renal failure
Surgically curable forms of hypertension
Benign resectable tumors of the brain or spinal cord
Heart failure due to arteriovenous fistulas or other high
   output states
Sepsis
Mechanical intestinal obstruction
Ruptured viscus
Subdural hematoma
Hyperparathyroidism
Hypoglycemia, especially that due to hyperinsulinism
Mechanical pulmonary obstruction

Add others as you learn about them . . .

207 Learn to trust your feelings. They can tell you a lot about the emotional state of your patients.

If you feel depressed, the patient may be depressed.

If you feel confused, the patient may be confused or even demented.

208 When talking with partially deaf patients, put your stethoscope in their ears and talk into the bell.
They will appreciate your thoughtfulness even if they still cannot hear.

209 With severely ill men over 75 years of age who are hospitalized, the absence of one or both hands on their genitals is a grave prognostic sign.

210 Order a sed rate.
It is a useful test when used wisely.

| 211 | Use laboratory tests like a rifle not a shotgun . . . one shot at a time and with precision. |

| 212 | In practice, occasionally send the laboratory some water with yellow food coloring.
Label it "urine."
Let the laboratory know you will do this from time to time. |

| 213 | Factitious fever does not elevate the pulse rate. |

| 214 | Paired or butterfly-shaped bruises on the skin are caused by pinching and are usually self-inflicted. |

| 215 | Factitious skin lesions do not appear between the scapulae. |

| 216 | Factitious disease needs to be considered in all patients who are undiagnosed or who have unusual findings. |

| 217 | Be wary of patients who bring their own pillows, especially if they are satin. |

| 218 | Factitious disease can occur as a collaboration between two people: the patient and a friend, parent or spouse. |

| 219 | Don't get mad at your patients if they don't improve with your therapy.

Don't get mad at your patients because of their life style.

Don't get mad at your patients.

If you do, get some help. |

| 220 | You must learn to listen for the murmurs of aortic stenosis and mitral stenosis.
Both are easily missed.
Both are correctable lesions. |

**221** The localized murmur of mitral stenosis can be hidden under a quarter.

**222** Pyloric obstruction can be an elusive diagnosis.
It can present as constipation or just a feeling of fullness.
The classic symptom of vomiting is sometimes not present.

**223** Thyrotoxicosis without a palpable thyroid gland is rare. When this occurs think of exogenous intake of thyroid hormone.

**224** LIVER SIZE IN VERY OBESE PATIENTS

Put your stethoscope over the liver.

Begin scratching the skin with a key well below the costal margin.

Move the scratching key toward the costal margin.

When the scratching crosses the liver edge, you will hear it distinctly.

225 If difficult patients ask whether they should go to the Mayo or Cleveland or Oschner Clinic, show your wisdom and concern by referring them there.

226 Learn how often each patient needs to return to see you. Some patients require weekly visits, some monthly, and others quarterly or annually or even every two or three years.

There is no rule of thumb to help you decide this.

227 When you do not have a specific diagnosis and the patient is up and about and not seriously ill, be very careful that you do not make up a diagnosis of a disease that will come to haunt you later.

It is sometimes better to use physiologically descriptive terms or the names of symptoms in these situations rather than disease diagnoses.

228 Avoid "organ" talk.
   Do not ask
   "How is your colon?"
      or
   "Your stomach?"
      or
   "Your sinuses?"
      or
   "Your heart?"
      or
   any other organ.
   Ask how the patient feels.
Do not let patients use organ talk.
Patients know only how they feel or what they think.
Insist on a language of symptoms, feelings, and thoughts.

229 There are no brittle diabetics.
There are only brittle doctors.

230  If a patient talks about a diagnosis, ask about the diagnosis.

If a patient says, "It started as the 'flu.'"
You ask, "What was that 'flu' like?"

231  In analyzing a symptom, keep asking questions until you can
make a mental picture of the patient having the symptom.

Begin to imagine how it would feel to have the symptom.

If you cannot do this, you probably do not have an accurate
description of the symptom and should ask more questions
about its nature.

232  After you think you understand the nature of a symptom,
repeat what you think you have heard. Do this until the
patient agrees (with a nodding head) that you have understood
what the symptom feels like and under what circumstances
it occurs.

233    Threats rarely induce compliance.

234    Never point or shake your finger at a patient.
       If you do that, please stop it.
       If you do not know if you do it, ask a friend.
       If you do not have a friend, make one.

235    THE RESPONSE YOU GET IS THE MESSAGE YOU SEND

If a patient gets mad as you talk,
you said something that angered the patient.

If a patient laughs as you talk,
you said something that was funny to the patient.

If the patient cries as you talk,
you said something that was sad or upsetting to the patient.

If the patient begins to argue with you,
you said something argumentative to the patient.

236   If you do not like the behavior of another person, consider
      changing YOUR behavior.

237   If you find yourself being frequently surprised by the responses
      of patients, you may be sending double messages:

          One message with your words . . .

          A different message with your tone of voice . . .

          Another with your facial expression . . .

          Still another with your body posture . . .

      Only an audio-video tape of yourself will uncover this kind of
      problem.

238   The first step in effective communication is to gain the full
      attention of the other person.
      Sometimes this requires long periods of silence.

**239** If a person's eyes are moving as you talk,
he or she is not listening with full attention.

**240** It is impossible to think and listen simultaneously.
    Listen
    Think
    Listen
    Think

**241** Listening requires practice.

Learn to stop thinking.
Learn to listen.

Just listen.

**242** Unless you can repeat what another person says and have that
person nod agreement, you have not listened accurately.
Practice this until it becomes natural for you.

**243** Learn to get the full attention of your patients.
Learn to give them your full attention.

**244** Anger overlies fear.
Do not respond to anger defensively.
Find out what the patient fears.

**245** Be careful with labels.
They can be very difficult to remove.

**246** There is a time for action.
There is a time for no action.

**247** Much disease is self-inflicted, wittingly or not.

**248** Do not throw instruments.

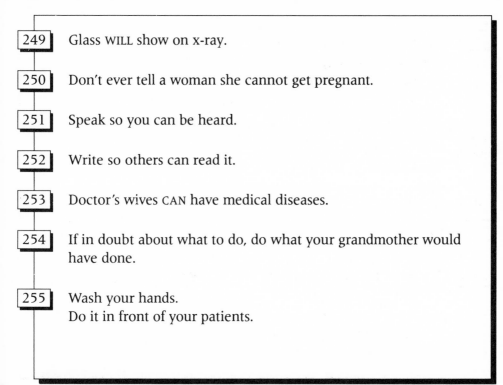

| 249 | Glass WILL show on x-ray. |
| 250 | Don't ever tell a woman she cannot get pregnant. |
| 251 | Speak so you can be heard. |
| 252 | Write so others can read it. |
| 253 | Doctor's wives CAN have medical diseases. |
| 254 | If in doubt about what to do, do what your grandmother would have done. |
| 255 | Wash your hands.<br>Do it in front of your patients. |

**256** Before you examine a patient:

> Warm your hands,
> Warm your stethoscope,
> And be sure to warm the speculum.

**257** When you don't know what to do,

> Do nothing!

**258** Do know harm.

> Do no harm.

**259** The brain needs a constant supply of oxygen and glucose.

**260** Restlessness can come from hypoxemia.
Go see old people who get restless at night.

| 261 | Enemas, sedatives, and use of multiple drugs cause nighttime falls. |

| 262 | Assume that the acute onset of confusion in an old person is infection. |

| 263 | Always observe the patient walking. |

| 264 | Unfortunately our entire system of health care too often teaches patients to stay sick, not to get well. |

| 265 | If there are difficult patients, then there are difficult physicians. We are of the same species, believe it or not. |

| 266 | A hospital is a dangerous place. Use it wisely and as briefly as possible. |

| 267 | No organ system fails in isolation. |

| 268 | Weigh every patient on admission to the hospital. |

| 269 | Weight gain or loss within 10 days is all water. |

| 270 | Be very kind to nurses.
They will be kind to you.

Be unkind to nurses.
They will make your life miserable. |

| 271 | Never tell a patient, "Don't worry." |

| 272 | The rules to make correct diagnoses in clinicopathological conferences (CPCs) apply only to CPCs. |

**273** THREE KINDS OF MEDICAL STUDENTS

The first student sees a bottle of red urine,
ignores it,
and pours it down the sink.

The second student sees a bottle of red urine,
wonders what causes the red color,
and pours it down the sink.

The third student sees a bottle of red urine,
wonders what causes the red color,
checks for red cells and finds none,
does a Watson-Schwartz test for porphobilinogen,
makes a diagnosis of porphyria,
and prevents an unnecessary emergency laparotomy.

**274** A bleeding scalp or facial laceration is never as bad it looks
initially.

| 275 | In the emergency room, assume that nothing is ever as bad as it looks at first. |
|---|---|
| 276 | Talk *with*, not *to* patients. |
| 277 | Never wake a patient to give a sedative or laxative. |
| 278 | If many medicines are used to treat a disease, none is effective. |
| 279 | Confusion is an essential phase of learning. |
| 280 | The first job of a physician is to determine if a patient is sick or well. |

| | If sick, what kind? |
|---|---|
| | If sick, how sick? |
| | If sick, what treatment? If any. |

281 The diagnostic process was not invented to determine if a patient is sick or well.

It was developed to determine what kind of sickness is present.

282 The assumption of a purely localized disease process in a systemic disease is a common error.

Here are some examples:
  Pericardial effusion in hypothyroidism
  Proteinuria in bacterial endocarditis
  Edema in hyperthyroidism
  Neurological deficits in pernicious anemia
  Embolic strokes from atrial thrombi
  Constipation in hypercalcemia
  Heart failure from anemia
  Dyspnea in hyperthyroidism

| 283 | Learn about the setting in which the disease developed. It will tell you much about the diagnosis. |

| 284 | The physician's belief determines the patient's belief. |

| 285 | Acquaintances of patients always tell terrifying stories about some person they knew who had the same disease, underwent the same operation, or who took the same drug as the patient.

They will always describe the worst possible outcome, complication, or reaction.

Warn your patients with new diagnoses of serious diseases that this will happen.

This will save you time. |

**286** There are more people taking thyroid hormone who do not need it than people taking it who do need it.

**287** If you doubt a drug will work, it probably will not.

**288** Only the patient knows how he or she feels.
No one else does.

**289** No suppository belongs in the nose.

**290** Silence raises anxiety.
Wait for the patient to break it.
The patient then will say something very important.

**291** A physician who treats himself has a fool for a patient
and a bigger fool for a physician.

**292** The error of making a false diagnosis of a nonexistent disease is hidden from all parties.

The patient is satisfied to have a name for the symptoms.
The physician has a diagnosis, albeit false.
The "disease" cannot progress since it does not exist.
The "disease" will always be a mild form.
The treatment will appear to work.

BE CAREFUL WITH LABELS . . . ESPECIALLY FALSE ONES.

**293** With chronic undiagnosed complaints, have the patient keep a symptom diary.

Look for correlations with activities, food, people, work, time, and location. Later you can add "thoughts."

If the symptom is said to be "constant," ask for hourly entries.
If the symptom is daily, ask for twice-a-day entries.
If the symptom is weekly or less, ask for daily entries.

**294** There are two assumptions that are helpful with any patient with a chronic illness:

The patient is doing something (albeit unconsciously) to aggravate the symptoms.

The patient is not doing something (albeit unconsciously) that would alleviate the symptoms.

**295** Ask patients with chronic symptoms two questions:

What are you *doing* that you should stop doing?
What are you *not doing* that you should be doing?

**296** All disease labels are abstractions.
Only the patient is concrete.

**297** Patients often take drugs from several physicians simultaneously.

298 Periodically have the patient or a family member bring in all the drugs the patient is taking.
With some ceremony, throw away any that can be stopped into a trash can.

299 Patients who are receiving money for disability rarely get well.

After the first year they never get well even if the money is less than they could earn working.

300 Once a physician and a patient agree on a diagnosis for a chronic disease, the disease becomes incurable.

BE CAREFUL WITH LABELS

301 Ask your patients what the specialist told them before you tell them what the specialist told you. This will save you and the patient a lot of confusion and re-explanations.

302 | Assume that unconscious patients (including those anesthetized) hear, understand, and will remember what you say.

303 | Reserve resuscitation for WITNESSED cardiac arrests.

304 | Stories and metaphors are wonderful teaching devices. To be effective, they must be closely related to the life and world of the patient:

Golf stories for golfers
Auto repair stories for mechanics
Computer analogies for accountants
Football or basketball games for sports fans
Fishing or hunting accounts for outdoor folks

305 | A few patients seem to be saying, "I want you to help me, but I won't let you."

**306** Learn to embed difficult questions in statements.

Instead of asking, "How much whisky do you drink a day?" Say, "I am wondering how much whisky you drink each day." Or, "I am wondering if whisky plays any role in your illness."

The patient will hear the statement as a question but not be threatened.

**307** Any lump found by a patient is probably more clinically significant than one found by a physician.

(An exception to this rule is the self-discovered calcified xiphoid process, sometimes reported in panic by middle-aged men as a tumor.)

**308** If an internist feels an ovary, it is probably diseased.

309　All recurring symptoms are triggered by something.
Find out what the trigger is.

310　You can usually ask questions about sensitive issues
on later interviews that you cannot ask on first interviews
(if you establish a relationship on the first interview).

311　If a patient takes a drug for several months,
he or she is on it for life,
unless a physician removes it.

312　Do not back out of the room as you are talking with the
patient.

313　If you add a drug, try to remove one.

**314** The last statement a patient makes as you leave the room is very important.

**315** Solving a difficult diagnostic puzzle requires the ability to study a workup and uncover what diseases were missed. You are looking for something that was not done or ordered.

This is a very different thought process from thinking about disease possibilities when working up a new patient.

**316** With very sick patients who are undiagnosed, think of poisoning.

Do this no matter what your impression of the family may be.

Test for poisoning before you discuss it with anyone.

**317** A careful and detailed occupational history can be helpful in diagnostic puzzles.

318    A detailed dietary history can be helpful diagnostically. Ask for details of what the patient ate at each meal over the past three days.

319    Do not miss protein malnutrition or dietary deficiency states. Obesity does not rule them out.

320    Find out who lives in the household with the patient.

321    Human emotional isolation is pathogenic and often lethal.

322    Be alert for hypnotic-sedative abuse, especially in old people. Withdrawal symptoms such as a seizure may be your first clue.

323    The error of missing a diagnosis of dementia in hospitalized patients is common. This occurs because cognitive mental status evaluations are too often omitted.

324 | The social persona is the last thing to be lost in dementia.
Do not be fooled by its preservation.
It does not take much brain power to be pleasant, sociable,
or carry on a rambling, but polite conversation.

Or even to act like the chairman of the board.

325 | Patients with dementia will do everything possible to hide
their disorientation, even to the reading of dates from
nearby milk cartons or newspapers when tested for
orientation.

326 | A test of orientation to time must include the day of the month,
the month, and THE YEAR.

Orientation to time can remain intact to everything except THE
YEAR.

**327** Always face the patient.
  Maintain eye contact that is comfortable to the patient.
  Do not stare.
  Some patients tolerate very little eye contact.
  Learn to observe out of the corner of your eye.

**328** Balance in life is essential.
  Pursue a hobby or some interest outside of medicine.

**329** The higher the technology, the greater the need for human contact.

**330** Your personal qualities can be as important therapeutically as any drug or treatment.

**331** After midnight all cases get clinically strange.

332    If you should inadvertently offend someone, say you are sorry and remember:

Everybody gets over everything, eventually.

333    Think of factitious disease when there are unusual findings, especially when caring for a physician's spouse or any health care worker.

334    The drugs taken by close relatives can be clues to some factitious diseases. Some examples are insulin, anticoagulants, digitoxin, quinidine.

335    Be wary of patients who say they have hypoglycemia and that nothing helps it.

336    Tell patients immediately when the subject arises that you do not believe in the chronic fatigue syndrome.

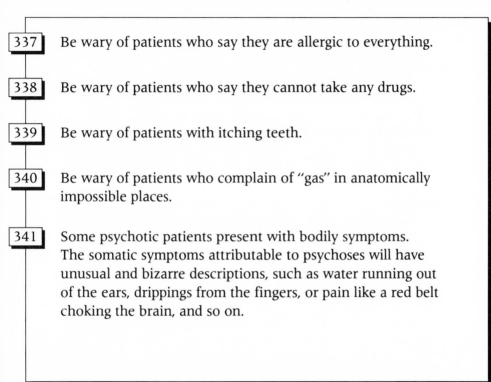

337 Be wary of patients who say they are allergic to everything.

338 Be wary of patients who say they cannot take any drugs.

339 Be wary of patients with itching teeth.

340 Be wary of patients who complain of "gas" in anatomically impossible places.

341 Some psychotic patients present with bodily symptoms. The somatic symptoms attributable to psychoses will have unusual and bizarre descriptions, such as water running out of the ears, drippings from the fingers, or pain like a red belt choking the brain, and so on.

FOR VERY ADVANCED STUDENTS

*Patients Who Say No Pain Medication Helps Them*

Try this with patients with chronic undiagnosed pain who say that no pain medication helps them. The patient must say this with an attitude that suggests pleasure in telling you this. It is essential that they have seen many physicians and that all have failed.

Carefully go through a list of all the non-narcotic pain relievers you would be willing to prescribe. Do this, slowly naming each drug one by one. As each is rejected, ask for details about why each particular drug cannot be taken.

After the patient has rejected all the pain relief drugs you know, you say, "We have established that there are no drugs that can help you. Where do you want to go from here?"

This approach gets all the drugs and drug conversation out of the way on the first visit. You are saying implicitly, "I have no drugs for you. That is settled."

Wait for the response and proceed accordingly.

343 Pay careful attention to patients who say they are going to die.

344 The first clue of dementia may be confusion at night.

345 A drug screen does not test for all known drugs.

346 Learn the difference between "informed persuasion" and "informed consent."

347 If you do something three times and it does not work, it will not work.

348 Physical distance and emotional distance between two people are not the same thing.

**349** There is an unconscious mind.

**350** It is more important to know the person with the disease than it is to know the disease.

**351** Masses are either palpable or not.
There is no such thing as a "suggestion of a mass."

**352** Do not confuse benign disorders with serious diseases and thereby expose patients to dangerous and unnecessary procedures.

**353** Never ignore an experienced nurse's observation.

**354** Patients with chronic neurological diseases always improve transiently when they change doctors or medications.

**355** Never leave the room while a patient is talking.

**356** Listen carefully when a patient prefaces a comment with, "This may not be important, but . . ."

**357** A doctor who takes a placebo to treat himself or herself has reached the lowest rung of the therapeutic ladder.

**358** On each return visit, ask patients to describe:

The color, size, and name of each pill or capsule . . .
The time of day they take each dose . . .
The number of each pill or capsule they take.

The few minutes it takes to hear this will save hours of problems later.

**359** Never ask a patient to do a favor for you.

Each physician is a drug.

With each encounter, a physician's actions can . . .

produce side effects . . .
exhibit a duration of action . . .
induce toxicity . . .
be indicated . . .
be contraindicated . . .
be given in an overdose . . .
be given in an underdose . . .
be given at the right interval . . .
be given at the wrong interval . . . or
most of all . . .

produce a placebo effect.

Learn the pharmacology of being a physician.

**361** Alcohol on the breath does not mean the patient is an alcoholic or even that he or she is intoxicated.

**362** Alcoholics can have serious medical diseases.

**363** A response to a placebo has no diagnostic significance.

Specifically it does not mean the patient is faking, or the pain is not real, or the patient is imagining some illness or symptom.

**364** Always leave a diagnostic loophole large enough to crawl back through.

**365** There is no substitute for direct observation.

**366** There is no substitute for data.

**367** Measure, measure, measure.
Observe, observe, observe.

**368** If you can't measure it, you can't treat it with drugs.

**369** Human perfectibility is an oxymoron.

**370** The level and intensity of care determine the characteristics
of the physician-patient relationship.

What would be paternalism and domineering behavior in the
outpatient setting can be appropriate care in an emergency.

No one in their right mind wants autonomy in an emergency
or critical care unit.

Personal autonomy returns with recovery from life-threatening
illness.

**371** The best prevention for malpractice is rapport with the patient and complete honesty.

**372** There are three stages of physician deterioration:

In the first stage, the physician tests for B12 levels and gives the vitamin only to patients with documented deficiencies.

In the second stage, the physician begins to give it to tired and weary patients whether or not they are deficient in vitamin B12.

In the third and final stage, the physician gives himself the vitamin.

**373** Be wary of patients who have had multiple surgical operations.

374 General questions produce informative answers.

"Tell me about your breathing."

Specific questions produce limited information and only yes or no answers.

"Have you ever had any shortness of breath?"

375 Read S.I. and A.R. Hayakawa's *Language in Thought and Action*.*

376 Be aware of and sensitive to natural losses in elderly persons: decreased hearing, poor appetite, loss of eyesight, difficulty sleeping, bowel irregularity.

Be sensitive to their psychological needs and symptoms: loneliness, depression, fear of being a burden, fear of death, loss of spouse, loss of friends, debilitation.

* Hayakawa SI, Hayakawa AR: Language in Thought and Action, 5th ed. San Diego, Harcourt Brace Jovanovich, 1991.

**377** Be wary of patients who bring packed suitcases to an office visit or the emergency room.

**378** Any behavior that is ignored will extinguish itself.

**379** A map of a territory is not the same as the territory. Do not confuse a model with reality.

**380** In medicine, anything that can happen will happen.

**381** Occasionally you can disarm a difficult patient with a compliment and make him or her your ally.

**382** Curiosity is not an indication for diagnostic testing. Curiosity kills not only cats but diagnostic accuracy.

383 Many patients do not change.
They just change doctors.

384 Use it or lose it.
This rule applies to all parts of the body.

385 The appendix is where the surgeon finds it.

386 The patient who is praying during the examination is probably gravely ill.

387 When talking to a large group of family members of an elderly man, all of whom are about the same age, you will find that the one with the largest hairdo is the new wife.
She is always standing alone.

388 Any procedure takes longer than the surgeon says it will.

389 A call from a nurse at night is always a plea for help.
Help should always be offered.

390 There is an old surgical saw that bleeding always stops.
However, it takes a real surgeon to stop all bleeding.

391 A consultant, above all else, is a teacher.

392 A symptom is a ticket the patient thinks he or she must have
punched to see you.

Listen behind the symptoms for the real reason the patient
comes to see you.

393 Tell people approaching old age: "Never start taking short
steps." It is a habit that can be avoided.

**394** Do not hasten death.
Do not prolong it needlessly.

**395** Surgery for poorly specified chronic abdominal pain will always result in permanent abdominal pain.

**396** Patients frequently do not take drugs as prescribed.

**397** No matter how much time you have spent in a patient's room explaining the condition, as you start to leave the family will ask one more question.

**398** Do not make the error of accepting the first abnormality found as the cause for the patient's symptoms.

**399** Good physicians are like good coaches.
They stay on the sidelines.
They never get in the game.

**400** Psychotherapy is sometimes like riding a well-trained horse down a familiar trail to a well-known destination.

The gentlest of pressure on the reins keeps the horse on the trail.

Only rarely is it necessary to pull.

**401** For most internal emotional states there is a visible and audible external representation in the face, body, and/or voice.

The astute physician learns to see and hear this.

**402** For unknown reasons, some patients have a tendency to insert all manner of foreign objects into their orifices.

The children go for those in the upper body . . . ears, nose, mouth, and trachea.

The adults go for those in the lower body . . . vagina, anus, urethra.

403 The mind readily sees and hears differences.
It takes concentration and effort to see or hear similarities.

404 There are several kinds of what is called noncompliance.

First, there are those patients who do not take your
prescribed drugs because they did not understand
the instructions.

Learn to communicate in their language.

Second, there are those patients who do not take your
recommended drugs because they do not trust your opinion.

Learn to build trust and respect.

Third, there are those patients who do not take your drugs
because they make them feel bad.

Learn to hear these people.
They are often correct.

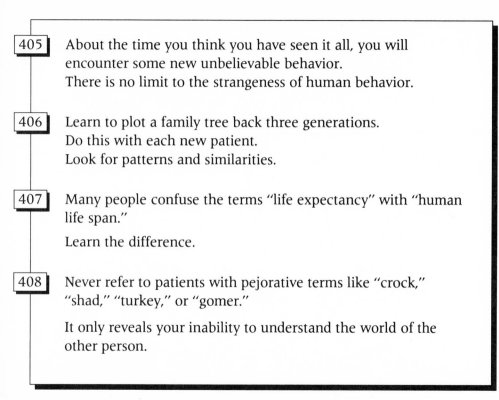

**405** About the time you think you have seen it all, you will encounter some new unbelievable behavior.

There is no limit to the strangeness of human behavior.

**406** Learn to plot a family tree back three generations.

Do this with each new patient.

Look for patterns and similarities.

**407** Many people confuse the terms "life expectancy" with "human life span."

Learn the difference.

**408** Never refer to patients with pejorative terms like "crock," "shad," "turkey," or "gomer."

It only reveals your inability to understand the world of the other person.

**409** No drug can be deemed to be completely worthless until it has been tried and shown to be ineffective in patients with scleroderma.

**410** Read Arthur J. Barsky's *Worried Sick.*\*

**411** The normal limits are not verities.
They are only statistically derived and defined terms.

Remember, at least 2.5% of the public live healthy and long lives well above the upper limits of any test.

Also remember, at least 2.5% of the public live healthy and long lives well below the lower limits of any test.

Everybody has to be somewhere.

\* Barsky AJ: Worried Sick. Boston, Little, Brown and Company, 1988.

412   Aesculapius is said to have spent most of his time keeping his
      two fighting daughters separated.

      One was Hygeia, the goddess of prevention.
      The other was Panacea, the goddess of cure.

413   The amount of external commotion at the death of a friend or
      family member is inversely proportional to the amount of
      genuine love and affection in life.

414   Read Thomas S. Kuhn's *Structure of a Scientific Revolution.**

415   The less often a patient has to take a medicine,
      the more likely he is to take each dose.

      * Kuhn TS: The Structure of a Scientific Revolution, 2nd ed. Chicago, University of
        Chicago Press, 1970.

**416** Be wary of hospitalized female patients with silver slippers.
Be careful of those with gold slippers.

**417** Language is the most important tool the physician has.
Learn to respect and use it wisely.

**418** If a patient is clearly lying to you, remember:

> The lie is usually addressed to "the doctor," not to you as a person.

> That fact, like the lie, are important medical symptoms.

> No patient lie should be held against the patient or get you angry.

**419** If a hospitalized patient doesn't want any more red Jell-O, get it stopped.

**420** There are three types of questions in clinical judgment:
The diagnostic question: What is wrong?
The therapeutic question: What can be done about it?
The ethical question: What should be done about it?

**421** You cannot diagnose what is not in your differential diagnosis.

**422** The four fundamental components of good clinical judgment:
Intelligence
Knowledge
Experience
Continuous critical analysis of results

**423** Read Eric Cassell's *The Nature of Suffering and the Goals of Medicine.**

---

* Cassell E: The Nature of Suffering and the Goals of Medicine. New York, Oxford University Press, 1991.

424    It is usually the second mistake in response to the first mistake that does the patient in.

425    Every era has its chronic fatigue syndrome equivalent:

> There was the soldier's heart in World War I;
> neurasthenia in the 1920s;
> reactive hypoglycemia in the 1930s and 40s, and again in the 70s;
> chronic brucellosis in the 1940s and 50s;
> and then there were retroverted uteruses and dropped kidneys and the ever-present and popular hiatal hernias.

We just have to face it.
Medical diseases cannot explain all of human misery.

There will always be a group of patients who do not feel good, tire easily, and need a large amount of rest.

Remember, everybody has to be something.

If you would like to suggest a rule for the next edition, please tear out or photocopy this page as many times as needed and submit to:

Clifton K. Meador, M.D.
c/o Hanley & Belfus, Inc.
210 South 13th Street
Philadelphia, PA 19107

Rule: _____

_____

_____

_____

_____

_____

From (name and address): _____

_____

_____